Six-Word Lessons to
PREPARE
FOR DYING

100 Lessons to Guide Those Who Are Dying and Those Who Journey Alongside Them

Amy Getter

Published by Pacelli Publishing
Bellevue, Washington

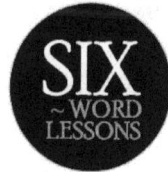

SIX
~WORD
LESSONS

Six-Word Lessons to Prepare for Dying

Published by Pacelli Publishing
9905 Lake Washington Blvd. NE, #D-103
Bellevue, Washington 98004
PacelliPublishing.com

Cover and interior designed by Pacelli Publishing
Cover image by Kyall McGee
Author photo by Chuck Getter

ISBN-10: 1-933750-95-2
ISBN-13: 978-1-933750-95-8

Testimonials

"Amy brilliantly takes her wealth of acquired knowledge of end-of-life care and distills it down. The format is very reachable and the language conversational. I hope that this is widely used to enhance knowledge and comfort during life's final journey." –Beth Turney, ARNP

"This book is wonderful! Bravo!" –Carolyn Jones, Award-winning Filmmaker, HOPE.film, CarolynJones.com

"This is a beautiful book and I am sure it will help many people, from those who are dying to those who care for them. Wisdom and love come shining clearly through the pages." –Karen Gerstenberger, Author of *Because of Katie*, Founder of *Katie's Comforters Guild* at Seattle Children's Hospital, KarenGerstenberger.com

Dedication

With love, for all my patients, friends and family
members who have so aptly demonstrated
this lesson:

*"You're braver than you believe, stronger
than you seem, and smarter than
you think."*

–A.A. Milne

Contents

Introduction

No one has all the answers for what is truly important, and what should be taken care of before reaching the end of life. This journey is individual for every person. But many who have known they had limited time remaining have approached their dying while taking some practical steps, both for easing the burden of their loved ones and providing for their own peace of mind. These 100 brief lessons are meant to offer some ideas, and prompt both awareness of and conversations about what might be important to you.

When You Find out You're Dying

1

Life will never be the same

You have received the news that the illness you have is not curable. You now live with a sense of the surreal: alternating between fantasy, such as "The doctor didn't really say that," and fact, screaming to yourself, "I'm going to die," when no one is around. What does someone do, when dying moves from the imagined to a real possibility?

2

There are no rules to this

No one has the "right way" or all the answers to journey through illness, and eventual dying. Just as every birth is a unique experience for every individual, the way you choose to go out of this life will be your own unique journey.

3

Try to have the hard conversations

Talking about your time left and your hopes and fears of what's ahead is hard to do. It might help to put things in writing that are important to you. Talk with those who will advocate for you. Choose the people you want to talk with, who will be on your team and support your wishes.

4

Your time is the right time

The right time to have difficult conversations is different for every person. You know your family and friends best, and you also know what you might not be able to manage at certain times. Speak up for yourself whenever you are able, and be sure you have a say in the timing of things whenever possible.

5

People don't mean it that way

You may be more sensitive than usual about many conversations that you hear, and although people mean well, they may share too much of their own stuff, or not even mention the obvious, or seem callous when they do mention it. Even though you are the one living with dying, try to give people grace—they often just don't know what to say.

6

Life isn't fair— today it sucks

Some days are like that. We all know life really isn't fair. Today, you might just want to spend time in the sadness. Give yourself permission to have days when you stay under the covers and refuse to join in.

7

Do you have a bucket list?

These are the things you haven't done, that you really hoped to do. Maybe you won't ascend the Himalayas, but that trip to the coast with family, or a weekend spent in Las Vegas with your spouse may be achievable for you. Do some things that you really want to now, while there is still time and energy for them.

8

Hoping for small and large miracles

Living with hope each step of the way can make days lighter and brighter. People outlive their predicted life expectancy all the time—after all, it's only an estimate, a best-guess. Keep hoping for things that are important to you, like more time, pain-free days, a happy birthday, living until the new year. Keep holding on to the goals you hope to achieve.

9

What matters most to you now?

This is a time of re-evaluating priorities. Do you know the things that matter the most to you now? You may want to practice the "six months to live" test. What would you do, where would you live, who would you be with if you had six months to live? Now is a good time to think this through.

From One Treatment to the Next

10

How to get
what you want

Start advocating for yourself! Not everyone is able to do this well, so you might need to rely on someone else to advocate for you. Have vital discussions with them now, to ensure they are supporting what is really important to you.

11

When a fighting chance means everything

Decisions must be made about what comes next, and sometimes you won't have a lot of time to think things through. You may be looking for any options, including clinical trials or experimental treatments, that might mean a promise of a few more months, or even beating the odds. Consider carefully the possibilities that are out there for you.

12

Is more always better than less?

Don't let others decide what you want for your life—unless you want them to make those decisions for you (and that's OK, too). Whether you say yes or no, don't feel coerced into making treatment choices— more isn't always better. Be sure the decisions represent what you want.

13

Know your options through the maze

In the maze of health care information, be sure you are truly informed. As your illness changes, the treatment plan will change, too. You will have to listen to a lot of medical jargon and sometimes difficult-to-understand explanations of various options. "Informed Consent" means you really understand what you are agreeing to.

14

Get to know what to expect

Ask questions! Keep a list! You won't know what is next without asking questions and getting answers. Make a list of questions to take with you to your appointments—you might have someone you trust take notes for you to refer to later on. As new questions arise, ask again!

15

"I like to be an ostrich"

You may not want to know, or you may need to stop the flow of information. You may not be the kind of person who wants all the information, all the time. Or you may be overwhelmed right now. Know yourself and know how you process information. Consider what has been helpful in the past dealing with difficulties, and practice that.

16

Become more of a rubber band

Having a life-threatening illness creates upheaval in every aspect of your life. You had things on the calendar, but woke up in the morning only to realize your plan for the day needs to be revised. Staying flexible can help reduce frustration when circumstances require a change of plans.

17

Can you whistle while you work?

The time will come when your job will become too difficult to manage. Find ways to use your energy and time well. Get help with accommodation for as long as possible, for as long as you want to continue working. Your human resources department's personnel and benefit specialists can help. Ask for advice on continuing insurance, accessing disability benefits, and financial planning assistance.

18

When there are children at home

As a parent, you may want to keep up the norm, doing the things that define your role as mother or father. You probably want to minimize the effect your illness has on your children. You'll need a good support system to help with this as you go through treatment. Work with both the medical staff and school staff to help point you in the direction of available resources.

Things That Can Help You Cope

19

When life doesn't seem worth living

Living with a life-threatening illness can create feelings of despair and depression. This is such a common experience that you will likely be screened for depression, and your doctor may recommend medication or other treatment for this. It's common for people to say, "I just want to be done," on days that are particularly hard to get through. Find people you can talk with about this.

20

Good self-care always makes sense

Set aside time to refuel and give yourself breaks. Do some positive self-talk, especially as you manage one day to the next. As much as you can, encourage habits in your daily life that make you feel better, for example: meditate, read a good book, plant flowers, nap, take a walk outside, spend time with family, eat healthy food, or go for a drive.

21

Positive thoughts to combat the negative

There is a lot to be said for the power of positive thinking. You can get help from others for this. Surround yourself with those who can encourage you, be your cheerleaders, and lift you up. Spend time with others who bring you joy.

22

"A happy heart is like medicine"

This quote is from Proverbs 17:22. Laughter is free, has no side effects, and can help you get through some very rough times. Remember to laugh a lot, whenever you can. There are many benefits to practicing optimism and humor!

23

Roles change—others can meet needs

You may have been the "little red hen" who did everything for everyone. You won't be able to keep this up, and in fact you will likely need to let go of this role, allowing others to help you now. You might be surprised at how well others in your life are able to do many things!

24

Cash in all your chips now

Now is the time for a return of favors. Try not to feel awkward if you must ask others for help, especially friends who have been on the receiving end from you, who may happily take this opportunity to do something in return.

25

Say yes more to offered help

People who are offering to help mean it. They want you to take them up on it. A calendar is very useful, letting friends and family sign up to help out with errands, meals, and other ways they can offer to do helpful tasks for you.

26

Your new phrase: "I'm bone tired"

Fatigue can result from the treatment phase you might be undergoing, and also may become a constant companion as illness progresses. Energy just seems to evaporate, especially toward the end of a day. Your energy will be limited, so try doing the things you want, at the time of day that is best for you.

27

The Nile River isn't always bad

There are times when "de-nile" can be useful. You may not be ready yet to face reality. You may even know this about yourself. Denial may be useful for you now. Don't let someone else insist that you "accept reality" if you are not in that space right now.

28

Doing good for yourself and others

Paying it forward can help you through the hard days ahead, such as being a cancer buddy to someone who has to navigate through their upcoming surgery and chemo treatments, volunteering at a community educational event, or joining a support group. Giving time to others going through a similar situation may add a sense of meaning and purpose to your days.

29

Recipes to help uplift and cope

Many cultures nurture loved ones with food, gathering together to enjoy meals and fellowship. A patient gave me their "coping recipe" years ago: Sharing a meal with a loving friend makes the day sweeter and brighter. Try meeting up with friends and lingering over tea and cookies a little longer.

30

Go out and live your life

My niece just marked her five-year survival of Stage 3-B breast cancer. Though she has been told that it isn't a matter of if, but when the cancer returns, she recently had an epiphany: Stop waiting for the other shoe to drop. Just go live today—now—fully.

Get the Help That You Want

31

Understanding the sum of every human

You are more than a compilation of bodily symptoms that are a result of this life-threatening illness. While you undergo various treatments and meet with medical personnel in settings that invade your privacy and personal space, you may feel like your physical body is the only thing they see, while your feelings and thoughts go unnoticed.

32

Nurturing the body, mind, and soul

Even the medical community recognizes that the mind, the body, and the soul must be nurtured (one reason for medical social workers and chaplains in hospitals). Connect with people to help manage the emotional and spiritual aspects of dying. These are just as relevant as how well your physical symptoms are cared for, and at times, one aspect may be more important to you than another.

33

"No more that can be done"

This is a nasty phrase to hear. In fact, though there may not be any treatment left that can cure your illness, there is always something to be done to keep you comfortable and provide quality time. Even if nothing may extend your days of life, a realistic goal for your medical team will be managing treatment to improve your quality of life each day.

34

Recognizing the time to let go

It's hard to let go, and realize that no matter how hard you fought, regardless of how hard you tried, a time will arrive, as you let go of more and more, that your dying becomes more of a reality. You may be overwhelmed with feelings such as sadness, anger, and resentment. Find people who can talk with you and help you understand your feelings.

35

When you can't do it yourself

How do you go about finding, requesting and accessing resources? Many medical clinics have a social worker or another designated person who can talk with you about community resources. You may want to consider outside help, such as a health care agency, or visiting nurse or hospice services.

36

What about hospice? The H-word

People misunderstand and shudder at the mention of hospice, thinking you "do hospice" at the very end of life. There are many reasons for not waiting until the final week of your life to consider hospice, especially for their encouragement, training, and available resources, including help that makes it possible for you to remain at home, if that is where you hope to die.

37

Hope never dies, it just changes

Your hope for a cure may not have been realized, but hope still exists. You can still hope for other things that can help you live the fullest, happiest and best life, which will help you have good days until you reach the end of your life.

38

Everyone hopes for a "good death"

What does this mean for you? A good death might mean extinguishing all pain, being surrounded by family, being totally unaware of what is happening to you, or retaining your consciousness to the very end. Consider what you want things to look like at the very end, and what is most important to you. Communicate your preferences to those you love.

39

"No one should die all alone"

Though this may be true for some, others don't want to be accompanied through their dying. Some very private people may not want family to care for them, nor anyone to witness their dying. In fact, they may wait until everyone leaves their room to breathe their last. Others may want to lie in the middle of the living room, witness to every minute of life. What do you want?

40

People who will be with you

Who do you hope to have care for you, who is important to you, and who do you want to be with you when you die? It may help to have conversations with these people. Are there some people you really do not want to come see you? This also should be discussed ahead of time.

41

Death with dignity, physician assisted suicide

If you are considering physician-assisted suicide, and it is legal in your state, know that it is a lengthy and expensive process. You will need time for completing paperwork and appointments with two separate physicians who will attest that your life expectancy is less than six months. One physician must agree to write the prescription and a pharmacy must agree to fill the prescription to hasten your death.

Living Your Life with New Symptoms

42

Talking and walking while chewing gum

As a life-limiting illness runs its natural course, you can expect that the abilities needed for taking care of business, getting around safely, going to the toilet, and getting adequate nutrition will all be affected. Although it is difficult to know when, performing these activities of daily living will become increasingly more difficult for you.

43

Yesterday I could do this myself

From one week to the next it may be more difficult to remain completely independent. Some solutions might be as simple as cooking meals in the microwave, or a wheelchair to move yourself from room to room. Talk to your medical team about finding options to keep doing things for yourself for as long as possible.

44

Have a "rainy day plan" ready

Just as you probably planned for your school choices, your career options, your partner, raising a family, and all other important aspects of life, you should begin planning for the time when you are not able to care for yourself, because this is inevitable at the end of your life. Make a "rainy day plan" now for changes that might suddenly make you unable to continue independently.

45

Symptoms come and symptoms may go

No one can perfectly predict how a disease progresses. You may have periods of reprieve, when symptoms are much less bothersome. Some symptoms, like pain, fatigue, nausea, difficulty breathing or sleeping, weakness, and swelling may need changes in medicines as they wax and wane. Always ask your medical team for help to lessen the burden of symptoms.

46

When you get all stuffed up

Constipation happens! There is a reason nurses are fixated on bowel care. Constipation contributes to pain, nausea, vomiting, and lack of appetite and it affects your quality of life. So, don't wait until you have a miserable belly ache, and can't go at all. You may need to take daily medication to stay regular. Talk with your doctor or nurse about this.

47

The 3 Fs: fruits, fluids, fiber

Try a few prunes every day, or drink a juice cocktail every morning, made of one-third each of orange, prune, and apple juice. For as long as possible, get daily exercise, eat healthy meals with a variety of fruits and vegetables, and drink plenty of fluids, although this can become an unrealistic goal in the last few weeks of life.

48

Fluids that aren't nice to mention

You likely have an entire row of medicine bottles that now live in your bathroom cabinet. GI Upset (gastrointestinal) listed in the medicine's side effects can easily alter your quality of life. Talk with your nurse or doctor about treatments used for nausea, vomiting, diarrhea, or constipation, and whether they will work for you.

49

What happens when you have pain

Don't wait until pain ruins your day. What level of pain are you happy with? Some diseases have a greater likelihood that opioid medicines will be necessary, but pain can often be helped by non-medicinal means, too, such as relaxation, massage, biofeedback, acupuncture, distraction, and music therapy, to name a few.

50

Some symptoms they don't talk about

There are common scenarios as death approaches that can be distressing to think about. Loss of independence is a natural part of dying, and you will likely become totally dependent on others for all your needs at some point. Incontinence is the inability to control your bladder or bowel. Will you want to have a catheter placed? You can talk about this with your nurse ahead of time.

Taking Care of Business: The Plan

51

Does it matter, once I die?

You might ask this question, and feel like there is little point in worrying about what happens later (after all, you won't be here). A simple thing to remember: some of your decision-making now can help make life a little easier for your loved ones later.

52

Legacies, legal matters, letters to write

Think about what you want to leave behind--things to see, hear, touch or ponder. There are many ways to create legacy for next generations, such as videos, audio tapes, written stories, and captioned pictures. Legacy for you might also be financial, and include ways to plan for future generations. Legacy might be as simple as writing a letter to loved ones, or future generations, to share your life lessons.

53

Writing your very own "death plan"

Expectant mothers often write a "birth plan," so that the things most important to them are considered during the time of birthing. Though everything may not go according to plan, what are the things you hope to have happen with your death plan? You may want to begin writing some things down, and start working on your plan now.

54

What do you need to do?

Keep in mind you will have less time, and less energy, as the days and weeks go by. Use your energy wisely, and say what needs to be said, do what needs to be done now. If you have a written plan, try checking a couple of things off your list each day until you feel like you are done.

55

How much planning is too much?

My mother-in-law, the day before her death, in response to a question about what to do with her things, answered, "They can fight about it when I'm gone." Everyone is different. You may have every aspect of your death-plan orchestrated, or wait and let somebody else make all or most of the decisions. It's your plan, so do it your way.

56

When children will survive their parent

One of the hardest things for a parent is knowing they will not be there for the future big moments. You can plan for upcoming events in your child's life, even though you won't actually be able to witness these things. You might write letters for each child, and purchase cards and gifts for future life events, with someone agreeing to share these with your growing children in the upcoming years.

57

Advance directives should be in advance

If you want to make your preferences known, including how much medical intervention you would want, and who should make decisions for you (if you can't), complete an advance directive now. This puts your wishes in writing. This means your family or doctors know your wishes if you are unable to participate in the decisions being considered.

58

Physician orders for life sustaining treatment

A POLST form (may be called MOLST or some other acronym) lists your choices for medical treatment if your heart or breathing stops. Would you want resuscitation efforts, mechanical ventilation, medically delivered nutrition, and other levels of medical intervention? Your doctor will sign the form with your choices, and you'll keep it at home to make your choices known, and prevent unwanted resuscitation efforts.

59

Writing a last will and testament

What happens to your "stuff" and how you want things to be dispersed among your loved ones can be clearly designated by writing a will. An estate lawyer may help with this. A written will may help ease the burden for family members, prevent issues after you're gone, and give you peace of mind.

60

It's less complicated than you think

You can write a will on anything, one of my patients used a napkin. Having the document notarized ensures that it was you who actually signed the document. If you are alone, or have only one beneficiary, you may just write down your wishes and put the paper in a safe place, as long as you have no concerns that what is written will be contested.

61

Not everyone intends completing a will

Some people may choose to not write a will, or simply not plan ahead at all. When this happens, and you die, you are considered "intestate," and the state decides who inherits from you. This usually follows a hierarchy of succession, if you have any living blood relatives.

62

Who are my next of kin?

The surviving spouse, adult children, parents, adult siblings, adult grand-children, grandparents, nieces, nephews, aunts, uncles, first cousins or other relatives in the descending order of blood relationship are usually considered next of kin. Check with your own state laws in terms of inheritance and decision-making.

What Does My Funeral Look Like?

63

What kind of question is that?

Choosing a funeral home and deciding on burial or cremation may seem morbid, but someone has to do it! Many people want to relieve their loved ones of making these arrangements. You can make pre-paid funeral plans, setting things up with a local funeral home, so family members can simply call the funeral home at the time of your death.

64

Deciding on cremation or a burial

Someone (you or a designated person, next of kin) must authorize the decision on cremation. You may want to choose the container used for the ashes. There are specific time frames and requirements for cremation and "green burials"—which means being left in a natural state and avoiding chemical embalming, so check with your funeral home for clarification and details.

65

What to write in my obituary?

Think about this question: "What do I hope they remember about me?" You may or may not want to write your own obituary, but you know best what things capture who you have been in your life, and the things that were important to you. Maybe just jot down a few items for your family to consider.

66

Who should officiate at my funeral?

This might be an easy choice for people who have a priest, rabbi, pastor or some other religious affiliation. If not, think about who might agree to participate and provide some time for that person to talk with you. Do they understand who you are, and the memorable moments for you in your life, and will they be able to share these things with others at your service?

67

Mates, music, musings, flowers, food, fun

Yes, just like folks make a list of guests, etc. for their wedding reception, you may want to take time to consider a number of things: people who should be "invited" to the funeral, (an address list can be helpful); favorite songs; who is asked to share/talk; favorite flowers to include; and what kinds of food and drink might be served. In other words, plan your wake!

68

How to plan an exit party

Some people chose to plan a "living wake," having a big party for all their relatives and friends before they die. If this is something you hope to do, you will need to plan ahead, and talk with family and friends to help make arrangements. Remember, because nobody really knows when you will die, you may not be present after all, or you may linger after attending your exit party!

What Happens When Death Comes Closer?

69

Dying is not for the faint-hearted

Dying is the hardest thing you will do. At times you will feel fearful, alone, and have tremendous worry about what the end will look like. Remember to be less self-reliant, and ask for support from family, church, friends, and medical personnel. Sharing the fears and worries you have may bring you some relief.

70

"I don't want to burden them"

You may feel increasingly concerned about burdening your loved ones. Over years of working with families who provided care to dying loved ones, I have heard many times, "I am so glad I could do this." It is a work of love to care for someone who is dying, and families share a great sense of satisfaction to be able to give this gift.

71

When you can't move from bed

Nearly everyone at some point near the end of life will spend hours to days or longer remaining in bed. There are many ways to make it easier to provide care for you in bed, such as positioning with pillows, having another pair of hands to help, and using a "draw sheet," to name a few. When dying at home, hospice provides invaluable training and help with this.

72

When transitioning from living to dying

At some point, you realize you aren't fighting to keep going anymore, and in fact begin to spiritually and mentally prepare—detaching from this life, and "turning inward," much like the metaphor of a caterpillar preparing a cocoon. This becomes a natural time of introspection with less energy for visiting, or caring for things you used to care about.

73

"How long?" or "Am I dying?"

This is a hard question to ask, and a harder question to answer. Some people simply want the validation—they know they are dying. No one really knows how long before you die, though we can watch for and often see signs that death is getting close.

74

When you know death is approaching

Many people have a sense that their time of death is drawing near. You may tell your family you think you are dying soon, and even have an idea of the specific day this will happen, or "choose" a special day that you won't die, such as a birthday or holiday.

75

Being able to say a goodbye

Perhaps you had hoped to see important people in your life one more time, to say goodbye, or you have a need to offer forgiveness or say, "I'm sorry," or you just want them to know how much you love them. Make the time for these visits now. When these loved ones are very distant from you, arrange a phone call, or Skype, or other means, to say goodbye.

76

What does death actually look like?

Many of the changes that occur toward the end of life have physical symptoms. Some common signs include appearing detached from this life and "turning inward," sleeping longer periods, episodes of confusion and anxiousness, and toward the very end, loss of consciousness, skin color and temperature changes, and rapid or slowed heart rate and breathing.

77

Not everyone has pain while dying

Nearly everyone worries about suffering pain. Some people have only mild pain, others may have times when pain is hard to deal with. Managing pain is a focus of care at the end of life. Opioid medications are often a part of controlling pain. You should tell your caregivers what level of pain you can tolerate, and what is OK with you.

78

"I just don't have an appetite"

Loss of appetite, no interest in eating, and feeling like food has no taste is common. Eating and digesting food takes effort. Try "drinking" your meals with smoothies, protein drinks, and milkshakes, and "grazing" your way through the day with frequent small bites. Try not to worry about the amount of food you take in. Usually several days before death, a person stops eating and drinking altogether.

The Last Few
Days of Life

79

As the body begins shutting down

All the organs in your body will become irreversibly less functional. Skin can be hot or cold, pale or flushed. Bowels are often not working at all. Shifts in blood levels of oxygen and nutrients affect all your body systems. Kidneys are less efficient with minimal, dark colored urine. Ineffective filtering in your blood and pumping of your heart can cause swelling in your extremities or your belly.

80

Comfort goals as death draws near

During these changes throughout your body, there is rarely any treatment that can be done to reverse this process of "body system failure" as death approaches. Usually the goals for your care will be focused on providing comfort and gentle care at the end of life.

81

Similarities of death and wax museums

Skin, as the body's largest organ, will undergo a number of changes toward the end of life. Skin slowly becomes thinner, dryer and paler and can be discolored (such as yellowish or greyish), having an almost see-through appearance. Pale, translucent and waxy-looking skin is often a hallmark of death drawing near.

82

Breathing may be hard to do

Changes in breathing are common when someone gets close to death. You might have slow, ragged irregular breathing, shallow, rapid stair-step breathing with periods of absent breaths, or deep, long breaths punctuated by no breaths. Though you may not be aware of any of these changes, others with you will notice.

83

Some call it the "death rattle"

This old phrase is used when describing respiratory congestion. It happens from losing the ability to swallow in the final days of life. Though sometimes hardly noticeable, this can worsen with wet-sounding breathing as fluid collects in the throat. Loud gurgling sounds can be hard to listen to. Sometimes turning side to side, and keeping the head of the bed up helps, and medicine may be used, but isn't always effective.

84

The colossal fear of the unknown

No one really knows what it's like to die, since no one comes back to tell us about it. Fear can be a part of anxiety and agitation that happens in the final days of your life. Sharing your fears might help lessen them. Physical changes in the body can contribute to anxious and restless behaviors at the end of life that may be controlled with regular doses of medication.

85

What does it mean to rally?

As death nears, you may be sleeping more and less aware, only taking sips of fluids, and seem to "fade away." Then a day arrives when you wake up, ask for a poached egg, and want to watch your favorite TV show. Your family may think you are getting better. Some people have a "rally day" in the last two or three days or week before death occurs.

86

What will my last words be?

Both mundane and amazing things are said as people die. You may tell someone you love them, or you may ask them to shut the door as they leave. You may not have great words of wisdom, or say anything monumental. Your family will remember, though.

87

Most don't die in their sleep

Most people have a slow trajectory of dying over a period of time, sometimes hours to days, sometimes days to weeks. Though after many days of increasing signs that death is nearing, someone may appear to just die in their sleep. In fact, dying took a longer period and the peaceful death that seemed like dying in their sleep occurred only in the final hours.

88

The death bed vigil for you

It is fairly unlikely you will be really cognizant of the "death bed vigil," but your family will always remember. You will most likely be in a semi-conscious or comatose state, and your loved ones will take turns sitting at your bedside, often speaking quietly and telling you remembrances, or visiting with each other as you lay dying.

89

I can still hear you now

My mother, as she lay dying, spoke words to me that I have never forgotten, before she reached the point of non-responsiveness so common at the end of life: "Honey, even when I can't answer you, I'll hear you and know you are there." I reminded everyone who came to see her of this—that she was listening.

90

If the dying could only talk

Here is what they might say: "Don't talk about me, or over me; talk to me, even if I can't respond. Guard my peace of mind. Allow the people I would want to be with me to stay. Protect me from the talkers, gawkers, and strident. Keep me clean and cared for, as you would hope to be. Provide dignity and compassion for me. Please, honor my wishes."

At the Time That Death Occurs

91

When you take your last breath

Your family may or may not be with you. Some people choose to die just after a loved one leaves the room. Even though your family may want to be there with you, and never leave your side for days, they may step away for only a few moments, and you may choose that very moment to breathe your last.

92

Do I really choose the timing?

Timing is a mysterious part of dying that no one can easily explain. It often seems as though the timing is significant, like right after someone says goodbye over the phone held to a dying person's ear, or following the moments a new baby is laid on the bed next to a dying person. You may even seem to be "holding on" until reaching a specific time.

93

Those last breaths may keep coming

Breathing can become so slowed that no one is really sure when the last moment happens. Some family members wait for many minutes, sometimes holding their own breath. A slow "last sigh" can happen a few times before breathing ends altogether.

94

After I am gone, what then?

If you are signed up with hospice, when you die at home your family simply calls the hospice number to report your death. There is no need to have 911 called, or have a medical examiner involved, as your death was an expected death while receiving hospice services.

95

There is nothing to hurry about

Once you have died, your family may need to take minutes or hours to feel ready to have the people from the funeral home arrive. They also may need to just sit with you for a time, or make calls to other loved ones to come over to sit with them. There is no need to hurry.

96

How to perform a death ritual

Whether ascribing to a religious or cultural affiliation or not, many people choose rituals to be performed at the time of death. These rituals could be: saying certain prayers, collecting flowers to lay over a loved one's body, singing favorite songs, performing a washing ceremony and dressing someone in special clothing, opening a window and burning candles, or lighting a bonfire, to name just a few.

97

Questions to answer after I'm gone

There are many practical aspects of death preparation that can help your loved ones. You might make a checklist with important phone numbers and addresses, provide access to financial documents (this helps determine the numbers of death certificates that will be needed), insurance, Medicare, Social Security, and others that can be filed for your family's use.

98

Signs that might be sent afterwards

Many people ask for a sign, after their loved one dies, to know their loved one is somehow still present, and that they are OK. Stories are told of bright moons rising, eagles flying overhead, double rainbows breaking through misty rain—some event giving a significant message for the loved ones left behind—letting them know that you are OK, and they will be OK, too.

99

Who remembers me when I'm gone?

Your loved ones remember you throughout their lifetimes, but next generations will have less to remember. Know that love lasts a lifetime, and some say beyond even that. Those you love and those who love you will keep a part of you in their hearts, always.

100

Are you really prepared to die?

My experience with death is watching from the sidelines. Most dying persons I've sat with appeared ready in their own way. Perhaps you'll feel ready, or have some things left undone. Find peace with yourself, if at all possible. "Be at peace with God, whatever you conceive him to be, and whatever your labors and aspirations, in the noisy confusion of life keep peace with your soul." --Max Ehrmann, Desiderata, 1952

About the Six-Word Lessons Series

Legend has it that Ernest Hemingway was challenged to write a story using only six words. He responded with the story, "For sale: baby shoes, never worn." The story tickles the imagination. Why were the shoes never worn? The answers are left up to the reader's imagination.

This style of writing has a number of aliases: postcard fiction, flash fiction, and micro fiction. Lonnie Pacelli was introduced to this concept in 2009 by a friend, and started thinking about how this extreme brevity could apply to today's communication culture of text messages, tweets and Facebook posts. He wrote the first book, *Six-Word Lessons for Project Managers*, then he and his wife Patty started helping other authors write and publish their own books in the series.

The books all have six-word chapters with six-word lesson titles, each followed by a one-page description. They can be written by entrepreneurs who want to promote their businesses, or anyone with a message to share.

See the entire ***Six-Word Lessons Series*** at **6wordlessons.com**